CW00848022

# HOMEOPATHY 101

## HOW YOU AND YOUR LOVED ONES CAN LIVE HAPPY, PAIN-FREE LIVES WITHOUT SIDE EFFECTS, USING HOMEOPATHIC MEDICINE

Polly Tomlinson

ISBN-13: 978-1-729328-41-5

# Contents

# Chapter *1*

## The Reasons for Writing This Book

The reason I decided to write this book is because although Homeopathy is used by over 500 million people worldwide with great success, only 10% of people in the UK use homeopathy currently, an estimated 6 million people.

*'O mickle is the powerful grace that lies in herbs, plants, stones, and their true qualities'.*

Romeo and Juliet II, 3

As a homeopath and healer, I am passionate about inspiring people to take control of their health and I promise that if you remain open to the ideas that will be presented in this book then you will discover a new way to approach your own health whilst feeling empowered to do so.

This book will stretch you and challenge you and it may even contradict some of what you have been brought up to believe.

What you will discover is not a traditional approach of modern medicine which we have been led to believe has a pill for every ill, and now know to be untrue, but a complementary medicine which yields amazing results whilst being safe, gentle and effective.

I can say with confidence, and no this is not arrogance, that this is a complete and true form of medicine, as after treating hundreds of patients I have seen so many flourish and improve their health in body, mind and spirit.

If you are fed up with a condition that you have been taking medication for and not getting the results you would like then this book is for you.

If you are suffering with side effects from a standard type of treatment for an illness then this book is also for you.

If you have tried all options offered to you without success, then this book is for you.

Or if you have already decided that you would like to embrace an alternative, then this book is for you.

If however you are happy with your current state, and resigned to the level of wellness you feel then this book is not for you, as you will be shown how to restore your body to health.

If you are ready to take the next step towards your own best health then this book is for you.

This book will change not only the way you view dis-ease in the body, but tell you about how this can be addressed using homeopathic methods.

All I ask of you at this stage is to be open to new ideas that may change your thought processes and how you do things from now on.

Homeopathic medicines are safe to use as they rarely cause side-effects. This means when used appropriately under the guidance of a qualified homeopath they can be taken by people of all ages, including babies, children and pregnant or breastfeeding women as well as the elderly.

Perhaps you keep getting colds, coughs, chest infections, asthma, allergic reactions or other acute illnesses and feel that your immune system is compromised.

Perhaps you are someone who has an illness and this is a long-term chronic condition which is showing little or no signs of improvement.

Perhaps you have an auto-immune disease and you have no idea how to get your body to heal itself rather than attack.

Or maybe you are a mother who would like to treat her children without using drugs for a condition, for example, eczema, asthma, colic, diarrhoea, ...and would like to keep the little one as pure as possible.

Or maybe as a mother, you have symptoms which require attention yourself. You may be trying to become pregnant, be pregnant, approaching labour or have a newborn and not wish to take drugs, especially if you are breast feeding.

Or maybe you are struggling with your emotions, suffering with anxiety, stress, or depression, or with PMT/hormone imbalances or mood swings.

If any of these scenarios are resonating with you, even if I have not yet mentioned your particular set of circumstances, and you would like to feel better, naturally and safely, then this book is for you.

If you would like to be restored to health, feel amazing, vibrant and full of energy, having eliminated your symptoms which are the effects of the disturbance in your body, then homeopathy is for you.

In this short book, I have written about what homeopathy is along with its philosophy, and I question is homeopathy for you and your condition, and can it work for you? I hope that the 101 questions which I answer in the body of the book answer the questions that you want to ask and dispel any myths you may have been told about homeopathy.

Imagine how you would be in your life if right now you could access this perfect state of health. Consider how you would be, how happy you would feel, how active you would be and how fulfilled you would feel with this new lifestyle. Imagine the increased energy levels, restorative sleep and mental well-being. This is all within your reach right now.

We all know that we should practise a healthy lifestyle and get into healthy habits including exercise, eating well and avoiding things that harm us, but have you ever considered what this actually means to you? Once you change your habits, your physical, emotional and mental health improves and these changes can have many benefits on your life.

Tina Turner wrote in her autobiography:

*'Life in the fast lane wore me down, changes in my diet and homeopathy saved me'.*

These new habits can help you to maintain a healthy weight and a healthy mood to boot. This enhanced mood, helps to reduce stress and keeps you fitter and more inclined to spend quality time with your friends and family.

Healthy habits ultimately help to prevent so many illnesses including heart disease, stroke, high blood pressure, diabetes, depression and arthritis to name a few. The bottom line is that this can give you more time on this Earth. More time to spend with your family, more energy to play and run around with your grandchildren perhaps or even to take part in extreme sports! Time to really enjoy your retirement, and watch your children and grandchildren grow up.

Getting better is not necessarily easy, but it is always worth it. Some habits are hard to break, but once you have and are feeling the benefits of a healthier lifestyle then you certainly won't regret it. Allow yourself some time to make these adjustments and stick to your plan and you will soon be feeling amazing!!

In the next chapter I would like to tell you a little about how I became a homeopath and why I am so passionate about helping people become their best selves by choosing healthy life choices.

# Chapter *2*

## My Story

To introduce myself, it might be helpful for you to have an idea about who I am and what made me become a homeopath and healer.

I grew up in a fairly rough part of north Liverpool in the UK. I was brought up by my mother alone who was a strong lady with high standards. Although we had little or no money, she always made sure that myself and my younger sister were well dressed in mainly hand-me-downs, and well-fed. My mother was one of the few people on our estate who would buy fresh fruit and veg, and flour to make bread. She put up with a lot of abuse on the estate but she showed me how to be strong and to stick to your beliefs. She always kept her head high when no doubt she was struggling.

She was a very caring woman as well and she was involved in teaching adults to read and was really involved in the local church.

Once my sister and I were old enough to walk home from school and let ourselves in to our flat, my Mum got a job in a local shop to earn some more money to live on. At some point, I can't remember exactly when, she managed to buy a piano and I would fall asleep listening to her play beautiful classical music in the evenings.

Later she began playing the organ at church every Sunday, as well as at funerals and weddings, and so the three of us would spend most of our Sunday there, firstly setting up for the service, taking part in the service, clearing up and then getting involved in the Sunday lunch which was for all the congregation. I had the job of collecting the money from all those staying for a three-course dinner in the church hall. Then we would all share the washing up. It was a real community spirit and we genuinely felt part of the church family.

However, Mum was depressed and as a child I could not understand why she was so unhappy and did not want to be here. She was taking a lot of tranquillisers and she attempted to take her own life on more than a few occasions. Afterwards, my sister and I would spend time staying with one family friend or another, and even the vicar and his family at one point.

I remember one night when she was in bed and I was around seven years old, I went in to kiss my Mum goodnight and she told me that she loved me but she would not be waking up in the morning. I left the bedroom confused and did not know what to do. She survived, but was hospitalised again.

When Mum was 33 and I was 10, she was diagnosed with breast cancer and had a full mastectomy. She was then put on a drug called Tamoxifen and took this for at least five years. Seemingly, Mum had the all-clear although she was never happy again really. I remember her buying lots of very frilly and flowery clothes to make herself feel womanly. She didn't have reconstruction surgery as it wasn't really on offer in those days.

A few years later when Mum was putting washing out on the line, a rib snapped! It was a shock and tests soon confirmed that she had bone and lymph cancer. So, the usual treatment commenced and she became more and more ill. Without going into the details, the radiotherapy did so much damage that my Mum died aged 42 at home.

But while Mum was ill this time around, she had turned to her beliefs more and I experienced some pretty amazing things with her. She was part of a healing missionary led by a Monsignor Michael Buckley who would do a healing service in the church and travelled extensively with his assistants, one of whom became my Mum. So, one week we might be in Blackpool and another in Wales somewhere with Michael who would do his thing in the church. Whether you believe in spiritual healing or not, it was an experience I will never forget. He would walk over to someone in the congregation, tell them what was wrong with them without asking and then lay his hands on them and pray. I once saw him call out a lady and tell her she was dying of a broken heart only to find out later that her husband had very recently died.

During one of these services, my Mum got up in the pulpit to give a testimony. I had no idea what she was going to say. Of all of the things she did say, the part that stuck with me was, 'If my Father wants me to be with him in heaven then so be it, I am ready'.

I wasn't ready!! I was very cross about her acceptance of her death soon approaching. We continued to argue about this on and off until she died. I was scared, and perhaps so was she, but she kept reminding me that if there is no quality of life then what is the point, that she had made her peace with everyone including God and she was ready to go.

During the next 10 years, of course a lot of things happened. I left home, met my husband and began a family of my own.

I shall fast forward here to 1998 when I am married with my second daughter who is around 18 months old and who has horrendous eczema.

I was in the throws of getting her the usual treatments and had been applying creams for some time. But she was not getting any better and her moods were also deteriorating. She would become really difficult to handle with tantrums etc., and her skin would flare up. I could see this happening in a cyclical fashion but I wasn't entirely sure which came first, the moods or the skin.

I decided to discuss this with my GP at the next appointment. I told him my quandary to which he replied, don't be ridiculous, body and mind are not connected.

What! Of course, they are! (screaming in my head).

I was really cross and right then decided I was going to find another way to deal with this dis-ease going on in my daughter's little body.

Amazingly, a few weeks later a clinic opened fairly near to me which I caught sight of and it was a homeopathic clinic. I had not had any experience of homeopathy (or so I thought) but I decided to give it a go and booked an appointment.

I learned so much about treating the illness from within, not suppressing symptoms and how to help the body heal during the time my daughter was being treated that I was hooked. I had found a medicine that did no harm, worked on the body and the mind and cured her within three months.

What was so interesting was that the first time I was handed the little homeopathic pills, I remembered I had seen these pills before. In fact, I had taken them before myself. I remembered my Mum taking me to an Indian doctor in Liverpool somewhere and him prescribing a homeopathic remedy for me in my teens. It all felt meant to be. My mum had opened my mind to body/mind/spirit healing and alternative medicine already.

When a friend of mine was suffering with the shock of hearing her fiancé had been killed, I tentatively went to see her with a homeopathic remedy. The doctor wanted her to take diazepam but that was not what she wanted. She did want the homeopathy however when I offered it to her and it really helped her. I was seeing homeopathy work in all areas of life and on the emotional plane as well as the mental and physical.

By this point I was very passionate about learning homeopathy, I was like a sponge and I studied for four years to qualify as a classical homeopath. I was delighted, if a bit zealous in those days when I was studying. I loved homeopathy and still do.

My sister had suffered with pompholyx eczema all her childhood and some of the treatment she had endured was simply barbaric, including the stripping of so many layers of her skin from her feet. For this she had to use crutches and only one foot was treated at a time so she could get around with her bandaged foot. Needless to say, she was one of my first patients and has no eczema at all these days.

Since qualifying, I have studied for a further four years to become a shamanic homeopath in addition to my classical training. I have had the pleasure of treating hundreds of people over the last nineteen years and I am as passionate today about homeopathy as I was then.

So now let's get to those questions you would like to ask in Homeopathy 101.

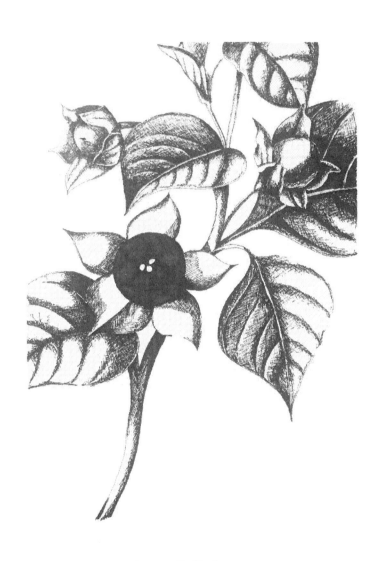

*Atropa Belladonna*

# Chapter *3*

## 101 Questions Answered

**Homeopathy easily explained**

1. What is homeopathy?

Homeopathy is a holistic medical therapy based on the teachings of Samuel Hahnemann. The primary rule of homeopathy is the Law of Similars which is used to treat ill people (and animals) with minute doses of substances.

2. Is homeopathy alternative or complementary?

In short, both. The definition of complementary/alternative medicine is something that is not taught at orthodox medical school and is not widely used by orthodox health care professionals.

Complementary medicine encompasses all health systems/modalities and practices which are not part of the dominant health care system.

3. What is the difference between homeopathy and allopathy? Allopathy is another name for orthodox medicine.

Allopathy is the treatment of disease using medicines or drugs whose effects are *different* from the disease being treated and have *no relationship* to the disease symptoms.

Allopathy is based on the Law of Opposites, (*contraria contrariis,*) as opposed to homeopathy which is based on the Law of Similars, (*simile similibus curentur,*) or 'like cures like'.

In orthodox medicine, illness is dealt with using surgery. Then a drug will be prescribed to counteract the effect of the symptoms and/or sometimes a drug will be given to replace something which the body is not producing any more, such as a hormone.

In allopathy, the action of the drug is what is required, not the action of the body.

As the effect of the drug reduces, more and more drugs are required, doses are increased and this can lead to a person developing a dependency on a drug.

Homeopathy treats illness and built-in constitutional problems by applying the 'like cures like' principle and using minute quantities of specially prepared substances.

These substances can be from a plant, animal or mineral kingdom. There is no reliance on drugs or dependency.

4. How does it work?

Homeopathic medicine stimulates the healing process within the body's own vital force and immune system and the body is restored to health all by itself. The result is independence from any medication and true health.

5. Is it safe?

Yes. Homeopathy is safe as it triggers the body into its own healing response. The remedies contain minimal doses of substances as opposed to orthodox drugs which may contain large material doses of chemical substances.

6. Is it effective?

Extremely! When the remedy is given, the reaction of the body is stimulated and the journey towards health begins.

7. Are there any contra-indications?

No. There is no reason why homeopathy cannot be administered to everyone.

8. Why is homeopathy preferable to other methods of medical practice?

Simply because of the things we have touched upon already. Homeopathy is safe. It is effective. There can be no dependency.

The homeopath's job is done when the patient has no more effects of illness and he/she is made redundant. This is the homeopaths mission, to let his/her patients go restored to full health.

9. Is homeopathy a placebo?

No. A placebo is an inert drug or substance given to satisfy patients. The word comes from the latin 'I shall please'. It was in the eighteenth century that the word placebo was used to mean a decoy drug.

The result of giving a placebo depends on the individual receiving it and their belief in the substance. Therefore, the outcome is determined by the person's interpretation. One study that tested the effectiveness of anti-depressant drugs showed that up to seventy five percent of the success rate was due to the placebo effect and that anti-depressants just don't work.

Some sceptics may refer to homeopathy as a placebo due to the dilution of the remedies, but this is not the case as the remedies contain the blueprint of the original substance within them. They are not simply sugar pills.

Homeopathic remedies contain very powerful minuscule doses of substances and are therefore not simply placebo.

10. Can I buy remedies without seeing a homeopath?

It may be possible to purchase homeopathic remedies from certain health food stores or pharmacies.

In my experience the potencies available are limited in shops and the staff have no more knowledge than the customer about homeopathy or which remedy to select.

You could purchase a remedy for say hay fever or a cold but this may or may not help as the remedy may not be the correct one for you based on your individual symptoms.

Unfortunately, this means that people tend to buy the wrong remedy to try, it doesn't work for them and then they have had a bad experience of homeopathy and decide that it does not work for them.

To achieve a true cure using homeopathy, the case of the individual must be taken by a professional homeopath and the bespoke remedy can then be selected.

For more information see
http://www.pollytomlinson.co.uk

11. Are homeopaths regulated?

There is no legal regulation of homeopathic practitioners in the UK. This means that anyone can practise as a homeopath, even if they have no qualifications or experience.

Voluntary regulation aims to protect patient safety and there are a number of professional associations that can help you find a homeopath who will practise the treatment in a way that's acceptable to you.

Always check that the homeopath you decide to visit is registered with a governing body accredited by the Professional Standards Authority.

I am a fully registered homeopath with the Alliance of Registered Homeopaths. For more information see www.a-r-h.org.

12. How much training does a homeopath undertake?

This depends on the homeopath and where they decide to study. For many of us it is a life long journey of continual learning and expanding of knowledge.

Personally, I have completed two, four-year diplomas in homeopathy and continue to attend post graduate training and seminars.

When you are as passionate about a subject as vast as homeopathy, every day there are new things to learn. I endeavour to use this knowledge when I spend time with my patients.

For more information see http://www.hchuk.com and http://www.shamanic-homoeopathy.com

13. How do I find a homeopath?

You may be introduced to a homeopath by a friend or family member who has found someone they trust and has had a great healing result. Recommendation is fantastic.

But maybe you can't get a referral or be recommended, if so then come and see me! www.pollytomlinson.co.uk

**What is The Philosophy of Homeopathy?**

14. When was homeopathy discovered?

Samuel Hahnemann first used the word 'homeopathy' ('homoios' in Greek means similar, 'pathos' means suffering) to refer to the principle of the Law of Similars in 1789.

15. Who discovered homeopathy?

Samuel Christian Hahnemann, born in Dresden, 1755 was a physician who practised medicine until the current practices of the day drove him away from medicine and he turned to translating for some years. He was a very intelligent man who could speak six languages as well as having studied medicine. He was also more than confident to speak his own mind and ask questions.

While he was translating an essay on herbs by a Dr Cullen from Edinburgh, he came across some writing about bark from the cinchona tree which contained a substance called quinine. He translated that quinine was an astringent herb that could heal malaria.
He was curious about this as why did this particular herb treat malaria and not more powerful astringents? A comment he added to the translation to Dr Cullen.

Hahnemann decided to investigate and took cinchona bark himself over a period of days whilst making meticulous notes of any symptoms he developed. Before taking the cinchona bark, he was a healthy person. Over the period of days, he developed fever, sweating, shivering and weakness, these are all the symptoms of malaria.

He wondered if this could be why this plant cured malaria as well.

16. What is a drug proving?

Fascinated by his initial findings, Hahnemann decided to repeat the cinchona bark tests which he called 'provings' on his acquaintances. He again noted their every response.

He then progressed onto other substances which were currently used widely in medicine such as arsenic, belladonna, and mercury.

The people involved had to be healthy, of sound body and mind and they could not take anything which may interfere with the results such as coffee, alcohol, tea or spicy food.

When looking at the results, Hahnemann saw some variation. In some cases, all the people involved developed a same symptom, Hahnemann called these key note symptoms. If less people developed a certain symptom then this would be classed as a second line symptom and the less common symptoms were classed as third line.

17. How was homeopathy put into a system of medicine?

Using the results of the provings, Hahnemann took the next step of using his medicines to treat sick people.

Before he gave a remedy, he questioned them about their life, health, attitude and examined them as well. He used these profiles to match symptoms as closely as possible to the proving picture of a particular substance. The closer the match, the better the results. He was beginning to see how like cures like in action.

However, there were some complications as some patients were showing aggravations or getting worse before they got better. In an attempt to rectify this, Hahnemann began to dilute his remedies.

First, he would make a mother tincture. Then he added 1 drop of this tincture to 99 drops of alcohol and shook the mixture by banging it a specific number of times on a hard-back book. This process was repeated as many times as necessary to reduce the aggravation in his patients.

18. What about Hippocrates?

Actually, the Law of Similars was previously described by Hippocrates and Paracelsus and was utilized by many cultures, including the Mayans, Chinese, Greeks, Native American Indians, and Asian Indians, but it was Hahnemann who put the Law of Similars into a systematic medical science.

Known as the father of medicine, Hippocrates (460-377 BC) stated, *'By similar things a disease is produced and through the application of the like is cured'.*

19. What is the homeopaths' mission?

In the Organon of Medicine written by Hahnemann the first piece of text states *'The sole mission of the physician is to cure rapidly, gently, permanently'.*

All homeopaths should be on this mission to restore health to the sick.

20. What is the Law of Similars?

The Law of Similars is a natural law which homeopaths follow when they are prescribing remedies. Sometimes expressed as 'like cures like,' this law enables a homeopath to correct symptoms of ill health with substances that produce similar symptoms when tested on a healthy person.

A very simple example of this to help you understand this principle is the use of homeopathic coffee called Coffea Cruda.

As you know coffee has strong effects on the body of a healthy person and for those most sensitive to it these effects can include palpitations, shaking, sweating, increased visits to the toilet, excitability, racing thoughts and sleeplessness.

Used homoeopathically, Coffea Cruda will relieve these same symptoms in someone who is unwell.

For example, someone suffering from insomnia caused by racing thoughts and the frequent need to visit the bathroom, might be prescribed Coffea Cruda.

As is it a Law of Similars and not exacts, it is only necessary for some of the symptoms to be present for the homeopathic remedy to work.

21. What is the Law of Cure?

The Law of Cure was devised in main by Dr. Constantine Hering who was the physician who introduced homeopathy to America.

Hering's Law states that healing takes place from the top of the body downwards, from the inner to the outer parts of the body and from the most important to the least important organs. He also says that cure takes place in reverse order, so the symptom that appeared first will be the last to disappear.

This is something I have seen many times vividly when treating skin cases. Children who have developed eczema over a few years will see their skin improve in reverse and so the last place for it to go may well be the first place it appeared – usually on the wrists, in the creases of the elbows and behind the knees.

22. What is a maintaining cause?

A maintaining cause or an obstacle to cure, is anything which interferes with the ability of the vital force of the body to react to the remedy given or to even recognise it. Sometimes a maintaining cause can be something in the lifestyle of the person or it may be a dietary factor.

Common maintaining causes are drugs which are powerful and can suppress the symptoms, suppress the immune system, create new symptoms or obscure what the body is trying to display.

Addictions, coffee, and self-medicating also create maintaining causes and must be addressed by the homeopath for a total cure to take place.

In these cases, the homeopath must give certain remedies to break through the drug layer which has been created.

Someone may be in a toxic or abusive relationship which interferes with their healing ability. These factors are all very important for the homeopath to consider before deciding to change a remedy.

23. What is suppression?

Homeopaths often talk about suppression. This is what happens when a disease is driven deeper into the body.

The simplest example of this is in skin disorders when the symptoms are removed/masked by the use of a medication, for example a steroid cream, which may well get rid of the symptoms for the time being.

However, this medicine has not dealt with the root cause of the problem and has just pushed the symptoms down until they reappear which they may well do. The more concerning problem is when diseases are deepened by suppression and a more serious illness can occur in the body.

*'A forcible concealment or masking of perceptible manifestations of a disease condition without the cure of the disease'.* S. Hahnemann, Organon of Medical Art

24. What is susceptibility?

This is the measure of how likely someone is to become ill when in contact with a disease. We do not always become ill because we are near someone who has a cold for example. This is when our susceptibility is low and our immune system is in good shape. Think about doctors and other medical staff who work with all kinds of contagious disease around them and never seem to become ill. These people have low susceptibility to disease.

Homeopathy aims to reduce a person's susceptibility to disease producing influences.

A homeopath may also comment if a patient is susceptible to a particular remedy if they have a really good strong reaction, or if perhaps they overreact a little with say an aggravation. (see 29.)

25. What is the vital force homeopaths refer to?

The vital force is the energy, force or power of the body which is able to overcome disease. The vital force varies from person to person and maintains life individually. Homeopaths consider the vital force to be a separate part of the being from the physical or chemical forces of the body.

In the Organon, Hahnemann wrote, *'In the healthy condition of man the Spirit-like Vital Force, the Dynamis that animates the material body, rules with unbounded sway and retains all the parts of the organism in admirable, harmonious, vital operation, as regards both sensations and functions, so that our indwelling, mason gifted mind can freely employ this living healthy instrument for the higher power of our existence'.*

26. What is succussion?

Homeopathic remedies are created using succussion as part of the process. This is the vigorous shaking with impact to potentise the remedy. Originally this was done by holding the vial of medicine in one hand, shaking it up and down and hitting it on a hard-backed book at least ten times. Nowadays this process is usually done by mechanical machines which succuss the remedies as they are being produced in the homeopathic pharmacy.

27. What is the memory of water?

The concept of the memory of water is of extreme importance to homeopathy as it may offer a scientific explanation of how high potency homeopathic remedies work.

The concept was first published by Professor Jacques Benveniste, in 1988, in the scientific journal Nature, where he claimed that water 'remembered' an antibody long after it was gone. At the time the discovery was met with much criticism.

Since then, science has continued to research the theory and is closer to discovering how the memory might relate to homeopathy. Current evidence is bringing us closer to explaining how homeopathy and the memory of water is a reality.

'There is strong evidence concerning many ways in which the mechanism of this 'memory' may come about. There are also mechanisms by which such solutions may possess effects on biological systems which substantially differ from plain water'. Professor Martin Chaplin of the Department of Applied Science at London Southbank University.

28. What is the difference between acute and chronic disease?

Homeopaths often refer to a case as being acute or chronic. Acute conditions are short in time, usually spanning days or weeks, may be rapid in onset and ending with either recovery or death. Examples are conditions such as a cold, flu, pneumonia, ear infection, bacterial infection and viral conditions such as chicken pox or measles. First aid conditions and injuries are acute initially, although they may become chronic if not well treated.

Untreated chronic conditions tend to become worse and worse as time goes by, without recovery, causing discomfort, pain, incapacity, or even death. Some viral infections such as herpes and AIDS are chronic diseases.

Many of the conditions I am asked to treat are chronic, such as diabetes, arthritis, eczema, allergies, auto immune diseases, endocrine/hormone dysfunction, asthma, heart disease and cancer symptoms.

29. What is an aggravation?

A homeopathic aggravation is when the patient feels worse or some of the symptoms get a little worse.

This can sometimes happen at the beginning of treatment and is a good sign, as it means the vital force has been stimulated by the remedy. The aggravation is always most dramatic in the first few days and then subsides as the patient is improving.

Homeopaths see this happening regularly as sometimes old symptoms have been suppressed with other treatments or medication and subsequently, these old symptoms surface as the cure is taking place.

This is simply an aggravation of symptoms as the person is getting better, it is not an aggravation of the disease/illness as the person feels better even with this aggravation. It should be said that an aggravation does not always occur, and this can be discussed when treatment with homeopathy is about to begin.

Personally, although aggravation is not a regular occurrence, I have treated many skin cases for example, where there has been an aggravation. This is generally after the prolonged use of steroid applications or other treatment that suppresses the skin condition. The aggravations which happen are always short lived and become less and less as homeopathic treatment continues. They are a great sign as the skin will never go back to how it was before and will continue to improve until a total cure is achieved.

**Is it for me?**

30. Can I take it while taking other medication?

Yes. It must be said that it is preferable to see patients displaying symptoms in their full-blown state, that is, not on medication, but this is not always possible.

Both young and old people are often on prescription drugs long-term and a large number of patients who come to me are already taking one or more drugs. This could be for example, a blood pressure drug, arthritis drug, statin, inhaler etc. These drugs are very commonly prescribed and so many people, particularly those who are a bit older may see their drugs as just part of their life.

Homeopaths are able to work alongside any medication as necessary.

31. Can I use homeopathy alongside other alternative treatments?

Homeopaths are able to work with patients who are using other alternative methods to help themselves and often this is the perfect thing for them to do.

It is common for patients to be seeing a therapist, counsellor or psychotherapist.

On a physical level they may see for example a physiotherapist, chiropractor or reflexologist whilst undergoing homeopathic treatment.

People who are working on themselves in any form for example Reiki, massage, shiatsu, meditation, acupuncture, etc., are clearly people committed to improving their quality of life. None of these treatments can interfere with the action of homeopathy.

One thing to note is that keeping essential oils too close to a remedy must be avoided as this can taint the remedy while in the bottle.

32. How long have you been ill?

The homeopath will ask you how long you have been ill as this is an indication of whether this is an acute case or a more deep or chronic condition that may take more managing. The homeopath will explain to you that if something has taken a number of years to manifest in the body then it will not take a few days to heal—or at least that is pretty unlikely.

Most patients appreciate this and so are ready to begin their journey and feel better daily.

33. Are you taking other medication?

The homeopath will ask this question to ascertain if there is a drug picture. This is the veil that can be seen when someone has their symptoms masked by a chemical drug in their body. Clearly the symptoms seen then are not the complete picture and the homeopath may need to work with what is there to begin treatment.

Personally, I have treated many people who have had such improvements that they have been able to reduce and ultimately stop taking a drug under their GP's supervision.

34. Does your prescribed medication improve your condition and well-being?

This is an interesting question as sometimes you may be taking a drug and not see any improvement. You may have been taking it and have got worse or you may be taking it and have no idea if it's helping or not, especially if you have been on it for a long time with repeat prescriptions.

35. Do you suffer with side effects?

You may be taking a drug and suffering with side effects which are creating more problems. All effects are effects where a chemical drug is concerned, side effects are simply the effects we are advised to ignore or put up with in my view. This explains why drugs can have a change of use when a 'side' effect becomes useful, for example using an anti-histamine for insomnia.

36. Who can it treat?

Everyone. Even the unborn child can be treated with homeopathy! I have had the pleasure of treating beings from the womb, through infancy and childhood, adulthood and old age. All ages can be treated with homeopathy.

## Homeopathy for Pregnancy, Labour, Infants, Children, First Aid & Our Pets

37. Can I have it while pregnant?

Yes, this is a wonderful time to give homeopathy. Homeopathy is perfectly safe and so the mother knows that she can take remedies without any side effects or danger to her baby. As the vital force is so strong during pregnancy, this is a marvellous time to treat the mother. Some of the symptoms presented are the baby's anyway and so by treating the mum, the baby is treated also.

Homeopaths like to give constitutional remedies to both parents prior to conception if possible and will advise a course of various tissue salt remedies to take in rotation while the baby is forming. This ensures that the mother does not get depleted in any way and stays in tip-top condition.

38. Can I take it while in labour?

Yes, and this can be an amazing experience for all involved. I have met midwives who have trained as homeopaths after seeing incredible things happen. The mothers who have these midwives on duty are very lucky.

I have attended a few births other than my own and have had the privilege of giving homeopathic remedies where needed. Remedies for the fear which may be present, or for the I can't do this, or for the I can't cope, or when the contractions are not as effective, efficient and regular as they should be.

In one case I gave a remedy as the medical staff went off to get the forceps trolley and the baby was being delivered by the time they came back! It was very quick and all perfect in the end.

Most homeopaths have an essential labour kit which can be made up and talked through with couples should they wish to use homeopathy during the birth. It is always good to make sure the birth partner knows how to use the remedies, more so than the mother.

For more information see www.pollytomlinson.co.uk

39. Can it be given to newborns?

Yes, it can, although most newborns are perfect and do not need any remedies at all.

If the mum is breastfeeding, then the baby will get everything needed through her milk. There are times when a remedy may be needed though, examples are shock from birth, jaundice, colic, diarrhoea, feeding problems, eczema, sleep problems, nappy rash, umbilical hernia, and for these conditions a remedy can be dropped on the baby's tongue.

40. Can it be given to children?

Absolutely yes. Treating children is so rewarding as when giving remedies to children there is usually little or no drug picture to get in the way of prescribing. Not only that, the strong vital force of a child will usually throw out some pretty spectacular symptoms. This makes it so clear which remedies are needed and in which potency too. To add to that, the results are quick as the vital force switches to restore balance once again. Beautiful!

Some of the common ailments presented to me are colds, diarrhoea, tummy bugs, conjunctivitis, fever, asthma, eczema, skin problems, sleep problems and vomiting.

As children get older their ailments develop and those most common are adenoids, asthma, ADHD, autism, bronchitis, chicken pox, measles, german measles, mumps, colds, coughs, constipation, epilepsy, fits, glue ear, lack of confidence, obesity, rashes, tantrums, worms, tonsillitis, toothache and whooping cough. It is a privilege and a very rewarding experience to see these children recover quickly with the correct homeopathic remedy.

41. Can it be used as first aid?

Certainly. I think most people have now heard of Arnica Montana, or Leopard's Bane and not without good reason. It is the number one remedy for trauma. Arnica can be given as a remedy after an accident to minimise the immediate effects of shocks, falls, bruising, bleeding and injuries caused by blunt objects. It also helps the traumatised tissues to heal.

There are a number of excellent first aid remedies which would be suggested for an emergency kit to have in the home.

Contact Polly for more information at
http://pollytomlinson.co.uk/contact-polly.html

42. Can it be given to pets or other animals?

It can and there are a number of homeopathic vets
in the UK. Otherwise, a homeopath can only
prescribe a remedy for your pet with your vet's
permission.

**What can it work for?**

43. What can it treat?

Homeopathic treatment is individualised and
focuses on the whole person rather than just
treating symptoms or disease names. So, for
example two people suffering from arthritis would
be unlikely to receive the same homeopathic
remedy because although they both have arthritis,
their symptoms may exhibit differently and their
character, lifestyle, anxiety levels, diet etc., would
be totally different.

Each case is therefore carefully considered and
treatment is specific to that person. For more
information see www.pollytomlinson.co.uk

**Physical, mental & emotional diseases**

44. Can physical diseases be treated?

Absolutely yes, they can. Your homeopath will take all your symptoms and discuss with you lots of things about yourself to find the correct remedy for you. It is very important with physical complaints to take the case carefully and to consider the sensations and feelings that are felt by the patient.

It is interesting that eczema is currently the most common referral to homeopathy by doctors. Other commonly treated complaints are chronic fatigue, menopausal disorder and osteoarthritis.

45. Can mental diseases be treated?

Yes, they certainly can. It may be that someone has no physical symptoms whatsoever and they are struggling with their mental health. A consultation with your homeopath will delve into how you are feeling, reacting, dealing with life as well as looking at your likes, dislikes, character and temperament. There are possibly the most remedies listed in the mind section of all homeopathic literature.

This does not mean that the homeopath cannot treat both physical and mental problems as often these come hand in hand. As usual, the case is taken in full and all aspects of you are treated. You are always treated as a whole, unlike conventional medicine which tends to look at us in parts.

Some of the most common symptoms are related to mental illnesses such as anxiety and panic disorders, bipolar disorder, depression, eating disorders, schizophrenia, substance abuse and addiction.

46. Can emotional diseases be treated?

Yes, as I touched upon in the earlier introductory chapters, one of my first experiences of homeopathy was dealing with a grief situation. There are so many emotional states which can be treated with homeopathy and the results are fantastic.

If you have an emotional problem homeopathy can help you.

Some of the examples of emotional disorders I have assisted with include the fear of abandonment, unstable relationships, unclear self-image, destructive behaviour, self-harm, mood swings and anger issues.

**Auto-immune diseases, pain and stress**

47. Can auto-immune diseases be treated?

An autoimmune disorder occurs when the body's immune system attacks and destroys healthy body tissue by mistake, but it can be resolved by homeopathic treatment.

When you have an autoimmune disorder, your immune system does not distinguish between healthy tissue and antigens. As a result, the body sets off a reaction that destroys normal tissues.

There are so many auto immune diseases including crohn's disease, graves disease/ hyperthyroidism, lupus, multiple sclerosis, psoriasis, rheumatoid arthritis, myasthenia gravis, thyroiditis, vitiligo to name a few from the list of over eighty diseases.

Homeopathy is extremely effective in treating autoimmune diseases. Homeopathy can help you to control or cure the autoimmune disease by stimulating the body to heal itself.

48. Can homeopathy help with pain?

Yes, homeopathy is very effective in treating pain. Unlike conventional medicine there is not a one-size-fits-all approach and so the type of pain is very important as well as when and where it occurs in the body.

The homeopath may ask you to describe your pain in detail. We all know pain is an unpleasant and uncomfortable sensation in the body. We also know it comes in varying degrees and maybe we can score it from a 1-10 to help describe it.

But we also need to consider is it a boring pain, burrowing, dull and steady, or is it say a cutting or darting pain, a digging pain or drawing pain, a lancinating, shooting, stitching pain usually sudden and sharp, or a sticking pain which feels like it pricks us.

All these descriptions will help the homeopath to prescribe the correct remedy to match your symptoms and so the more information she is given, the better the remedy selection will be.

49. Can homeopathy help with stress?

Stress in medical terms is different from anxiety and is caused by particular situations or events in your life that may make you feel frustrated, angry, worried or even anxious. The stress response is different for each individual and so the same event can often cause different responses in different people.

Some common causes of stress include public speaking, work deadlines, difficult family or friend circumstances, some social situations or changes in the work place.

As I have said already, homeopathy is effective because it is a holistic medicine that treats you as a whole and therefore treatment will include addressing the underlying issues that lead to stress. Homeopathy recognises the uniqueness of you and treats you accordingly.

Identifying the factors that cause stress, and the various reactions, are of vital importance in homeopathy since symptoms are most often manifested when you are exposed to an external force stronger than your internal vitality and immune system.

Therefore, treating symptoms superficially will only act as a temporary palliative and will not provide a lasting cure.

Homeopathy, aims to cure the underlying stress response and can permanently eliminate its symptoms.

The homeopath will consider many aspects including your mental/emotional state, the location of the symptoms, your behaviour towards the symptoms, susceptibility, family history, and more. This is then analysed allowing him/her to recognise underlying causes of stress or anxiety experienced by you, and to select a fitting remedy.

**Homeopathy for the elderly and adolescents**

50. What about problems in the elderly?

As we age, it is important to recognise that health is more likely to be maintained by being connected to family and friends or to the community in some way as well as being concerned with the workings of our bodies.

I feel very strongly that the use of homeopathy in the elderly can help you to avoid the use of multiple medications which become a way of life and create more problems in the long run. Older bodies can be less efficient at dealing with the processing of conventional medicines and so the side effects can be more serious and can build up over time.

Homeopathic medicines do not put any strain on the body, they are gentle as well as being effective.

Over the years, many layers of diseases may have built up in you and so good constitutional treatment is needed. The homeopath can prescribe the best remedies to improve both the quality of life in the sense of vitality and well-being, but also improve symptoms.

Some conditions which are commonly presented to homeopaths include confusion, depression, falls, accidents, dementia and skin problems.

51. What about problems in adolescents?

Adolescence is a time of great turmoil for many young people. Puberty usually begins from 10 years old in girls and 11 years old in boys. It is a time of emotional and intellectual change, where the individual really begins to feel the outside world and to react to it.

It is a time of finding some independence and it is the parents' job to 'spar' with them and set boundaries for them to push against. It can be a difficult time for all involved and no doubt brings up some tricky situations which cause conflict while everyone finds their new position in the dynamic of the family.

The young person is torn between wanting no responsibilities and wanting to be free and with his or her friends and being at home with their parents doing what they do. Depending on the type of parenting, this period of growth can be a difficult and lonely time for them.

Adolescents need loving no matter how they are behaving! Once they have some space for themselves and the parents are allowed some too, the healthy transition to adulthood is set to follow.

Homeopathy treats the individual as a whole person and listens to the needs and wants of the adolescent to ascertain which is the correct remedy to help them at this turning point in their life.

Some conditions which are commonly presented to homeopaths by adolescents include acne, anxiety due to exams or bullying for example, depression, drug addiction, food disorders, self-harm and puberty problems.

**Homeopathy for fertility, pregnancy, childbirth, for the mother and the infant**

52. What about fertility problems?

One of the most important reasons that someone comes to see a homeopath is to help them to conceive and have a healthy pregnancy and birth. Homeopathy can be a huge help and a constitutional remedy can have amazing results.

For couples who may have been trying for some time with no success, homeopathy can be a great discovery. Some couples come to a homeopath after having tried IVF treatment, others come before venturing along this route.

There is a great deal of physical and emotional turmoil in the situation. There may be physical issues which need to be addressed such as fibroids, endometriosis, blocked fallopian tubes, polycystic ovary syndrome, poor ovulation, poor egg or sperm quality.

Other blocks can be a result of the contraceptive pill or other contraception which has stopped the menstrual cycle for a long period of time. There may have been previous miscarriages, addiction, toxicity or emotional issues such as trauma or grief.

Homeopathy is safe and effective as well as being painless. The homeopath considers the whole person (and I like to treat both members of the couple where possible) and takes into account any potential blocks to fertility. Removal of these blocks using the remedies can often result in a healthy pregnancy.

Have you had any of the following problems: Been trying to conceive for over three months with no success, had previous miscarriage or grief situation, any emotional problems in your relationship, gynaecological problems, been given hormonal treatment? Then homeopathy can help.

53. What about problems in pregnancy and childbirth?

During pregnancy there may be no need for any medicines of any sort and this is advisable especially during the first three months.

Homeopathic tissue salts can be prescribed however and are very gentle. These remedies support the mother while the baby is growing and can help with common complaints such as stretch marks, general elasticity of the skin, iron deficiency, swollen ankles, indigestion and muscle cramps to name a few.

For other complaints, homeopathy is so effective. Some of the ailments I have encountered include back ache, anaemia, breech presentation, constipation, cramp, acid reflux, fainting, emotional disturbance, blood pressure, morning sickness and sleeping problems.

Excitingly, there are homeopathic remedies to help during labour and this I have experienced myself as well as at other births. The results are fantastic! I have seen a baby delivered in forty-five minutes while the nurses went away to fetch the forceps trolley!

The remedies can be made up in a kit and usually I would discuss the remedies with the birth partner as well as they will be in charge of administering the remedies at the right time. The remedies in the kit cover a wide variety of situations, feelings and emotions as well as physical difficulties such as ineffective contractions.

Homeopathy truly is amazing!

54. What about homeopathy for the infant and the mother?

The list of problems that homeopathy can help with is so helpful to the new mother and also the baby.

I have administered remedies to help after a C-section or stitches, for breastfeeding problems or mastitis, for after-pains, exhaustion, incontinence as well as post-natal depression.

Remedies also help with jaundice and in this instance if the mother is breastfeeding then she takes the remedy and nurses the baby. Beautiful!

**Homeopathic vaccination**

55. Are there homeopathic alternatives to vaccination?

Yes, there are. Homeopathic prophylaxis as it's called is very effective and there are many examples of its results which can be found in various homeopathic books.

An example is the remedy pertussin which is used when contact has been made with whooping cough, or simply as a homeopathic vaccination. In one outbreak of whooping cough three hundred and sixty-four children were given pertussin after contact with the disease and not one of them developed whooping cough.

In Cuba, in 2007, conventional medical researchers gave homeopathic leptospirosis prophylaxis to the population due to the desperate situation. They were overwhelmed by the disease after the hurricane season and had limited conventional resources. Basically, they had no other options and the homeopathic remedy could be produced in a very short period of time. The results were so successful there was a ninety percent decrease in the region (a region of 2.1 million people). The following year, the remedy was given to the whole population of eleven million people and the disease has now virtually been eradicated. This could have never been achieved with conventional medicine. Based on these results, the Cuban Ministry of Health now uses homeopathic prophylaxis for various epidemics including dengue fever, 'swine' flu, hepatitis A and conjunctivitis, all with success.

Homeopaths are able to use plant, animal and mineral remedies to protect against various diseases. They can also use nosodes which are remedies made from the actual diseased body tissue or sputum for example. These remedies are prepared in exactly the same way as the usual remedies and so there is no diseased tissue remaining in them when they are administered. Therefore, there is no risk of harm.

If you are considering vaccination and have decided that you would like to use an alternative then you need to contact your homeopath. I have experience of using alternatives to vaccination and nosodes to treat small babies, children, teenagers as well as adults who are advised to have a vaccination for example before travelling.

There are homeopathic prophylaxis for diseases from diphtheria, flu, malaria, measles, mumps, meningitis, polio, tetanus, rubella, tuberculosis, whooping cough and more being developed.

For more information see www.pollytomlinson.co.uk

**What should I expect?**

56. What does a homeopath do?

Essentially, I take your case by asking questions and listening in great detail to your story of what has happened to you, how you feel and what you need help with. I am always an unprejudiced observer, I have no preconceived ideas and I make no judgements. I have to maintain a clear mind to do my best work and I am most intrigued by the strange rare and peculiar things that come up when we talk.

I will do a lot of note taking while you talk, this is essential for me to analyse the case and select the correct remedy.

It is also useful for follow-on appointments when we can run through changes. I find that once a symptom has gone, you will forget that you even had it in the first place. This is great to see.

57. Can I have a consultation with a homeopath on the phone or via Skype?

Yes. This is now possible. When it is not possible for a patient to get to my clinic, I am happy to do a consultation by skype/phone/facetime etc., As long as we are both fully present and treating the session as if we were together then this will work perfectly well.

See http://www.pollytomlinson.co.uk/contact-polly.html

58. What should I expect at my first consultation?

At the first consultation there will be a lot of questions to answer. You will be asked about your illness, and how it affects you. You will be asked about your medical history from your mother's pregnancy onwards and about family history. You will also be asked about your likes and dislikes, appetite, diet, bodily functions, emotions and temperament. It is a detailed discussion and although some of the questions may seem irrelevant to you, they are helping the homeopath to build a picture of your constitutional type.

59. How is the case analysed?

When listening to you talk, you will reveal a great deal about yourself. This is done through speaking and body language. I will be observing and looking at what is being presented to me. I will be taking notes and all the information will be used to enable me to select the correct remedies.

60. How does a homeopath select the correct remedy?

When I am taking a case, a picture of one or more remedies may enter my head. Then the internal filtration system kicks in, in my mind which leads me to certain remedies which I have learned during training and through years of practice. I will look at these remedies in some Materia Medica books to confirm my decision making.

Some homeopaths have the knowledge of thousands of remedies while others work with a handful of important remedies that they know inside out. Some homeopaths like to use a computer system to calculate the remedy which is most appropriate, these are the ones who like technology, others like myself tend to use a handful of books and others none at all. There is no correct approach in my view as we are all aiming for a cure.

61. Where does the homeopath get the remedies from?

I purchase all my remedies from reputable homeopathic pharmacies in the UK. These pharmacies are licensed by both the Medicines and Healthcare Products Regulatory Agency (MHRA) and the

Veterinary Medicines Directorate (VMD). This ensures that they manufacture in accordance with a strict Quality Assurance Programme and Good Manufacturing Practice.

Pharmacies and suppliers include:
https://www.ainsworths.com,
https://www.helios.co.uk,
https://www.hsconline.co.uk/home

62. How does a homeopath select the correct potency?

So once the remedy or possible remedies have been selected, then the potency must be decided also. The highest potencies containing the least substance, can penetrate the most subtle levels of disease and so it is the homeopath's job to find the correct potency for you.

Very generally speaking, lower potencies are used for physical conditions whereas higher potencies delve into the realms of the mind, emotion and the spiritual.

63. How do I take a homeopathic remedy?

The remedies are generally made up as small pillules which are placed under the tongue to dissolve. If this is not possible for any reason remedies may be made up as liquids or powders to be poured onto the tongue (very useful for babies).

In India, homeopuncture combines the use of the remedy with the tip of the needle.

64. How often will I take the remedy?

This also depends on the symptoms and the constitution of the patient. Some remedies are taken often, a few times a day or even more frequent, every half an hour in an acute or emergency situation. In other cases, a remedy may be needed daily or it may be necessary to provide a few or just one dose. The homeopath will lead you always as to the best way to proceed for you.

65. How long will I need to take the remedy for?

Until there is a change in the symptoms and it is clear that your health is improving. I usually explain this to my patients using the analogy of jump starting a car. Once the car is running smoothly, and it may have taken a few attempts, then there is no need to keep on doing it. Just allow the car [body] to do its thing now as it builds up its strength once again.

66. How long will the treatment take?

In acute cases where for example there is a high temperature or say vomitting/diarrhoea, the correctly selected remedy can work within minutes.

In first aid situations where homeopathy is used after an accident the results can be really fast, for example after a burn, cut, bang or bruise, and other injuries.

However, if a patient has a chronic condition which has taken many years to manifest in the body then it is unlikely to be cured instantly. In this case it may take longer to get back to good health.

67. How long will the cure last?

Once the cure is reached then homeopathy has done its job and the body will remain well.

However, as we know there may be outside influences which could cause you to become ill again, these may be a maintaining cause such as an unhealthy relationship, addiction or a poor diet.

68. How will I know my treatment is working?

You will know your treatment is working when the symptoms begin to improve or if you have had some sort of aggravation of the symptoms when you began taking the remedy.

69. How will I feel?

You will feel well, vibrant, energy levels will be improved and you will know that your symptoms are improving as well.

70. What do I do if my symptoms change?

Your symptoms should change in terms of improvement. When this happens, it is time to stop the remedy and let the body continue its healing action.

If your symptoms change in terms of something different appearing it would be wise to discuss this with your homeopath. If the symptoms are old symptoms that you have experienced before, then this is a sign of cure following the Law of Cure which homeopaths follow. This often happens but the old symptoms generally appear in a very mild way as the body restores itself.

If the symptoms are completely new then there may be another reason for these and this should be discussed to determine whether a change of remedy is needed or whether the remedy should be stopped.

Your homeopath will know what to do and advise you accordingly.

71. Will my symptoms get worse before they get better?

Sometimes you may feel worse or some of the symptoms get a little worse for a short time.

This can sometimes happen at the beginning of treatment and is a good sign, as it means the vital force has been stimulated by the remedy. The aggravation is always most dramatic in the first few days and then subsides as the patient is improving.

Homeopaths see this happening regularly as sometimes old symptoms have been suppressed with other treatments or medication and subsequently, these old symptoms surface as the cure is taking place.

**What are the remedies and how do I take them?**

72. What are the remedies made from?

Homeopathic medicine is made from extremely small quantities of nanoparticles of substances extracted from plants, animals or minerals.

73. What are mother tinctures?

A mother tincture is made by adding the substance needed to alcohol and leaving this to stand for approximately a month. The liquid is then strained to produce the mother tincture itself. If the substance is insoluble then it is triturated, or ground up before being added to the solvent/alcohol.

74. How are the remedies prepared?

The remedies are prepared from the mother tincture of the substance, this is the starting point, a herbal tincture if it is made from a plant.

For the preparation of liquid potencies from solutions of soluble substances, triturates, or plant mother tincture, there is a two-part process at each step. First, a one to one hundred dilution of the solution is prepared and then this is succussed (shaken with impact) vigorously at each step. This is usually done mechanically with the same number of strokes and with the same force. This would result in a 1c potency. This is repeated to create 2c, 3c etc., until the desired potency is reached.

There are other scales of dilution used as well such as the x potencies which are diluted one to ten. All remedies are succussed at each stage, this is an imperative part of the process.

These liquid potencies are then used to medicate the little sugar pills that are given to you.

75. Why are there different potencies?

The different potencies prepared means that there are different amounts of the original substance and energy of the substance in the remedy depending on how high or low the potency is.

The homeopath has to select the correct remedy to match not only your symptoms but also your vitality. Hence the need for many potencies.

76. What are tissue salts?

Tissue salts were invented by the German doctor, Wilhelm Schuessler, who believed that ill health was caused by the imbalance of the twelve cell salts or minerals that make up our bodies.

He created these remedies in a 6x potency to enable the body to easily absorb the cell salts in homeopathic form, that is in micro doses. He believed that the remedies give the body all it needs to repair and maintain itself.

They are gentle and so able to be used by the very young as well as old, whilst pregnant and by your pets.

77. What are imponderabilia remedies?

Imponderabilia means that which is not weighable, i.e., the substances which have no perceptible weights, they are immaterial power or energy and they may be natural or artificial. Medicines prepared from energy, available from natural and physical reactions are called imponderabilia.

Hahnemann observed in his Organon that, *'even imponderable agencies can produce most violent effects upon man'.*

The first 'Imponderable' was proven by Hahnemann in 1833. In an era, rich with scientific experimentation and questioning, it is completely understandable that Hahnemann would be eager to prove natural phenomena, and his choice was magnetism.

In the last 100 years many imponderabilia remedies have been created using the energy from the moon, the sun, light from various planets and stars, mobile phones, computer games, x-ray, mri radiation, ultrasound, TV emanation, the colour spectrum, crystal energies and microwaves to name a few. The list is endless as technology forges ahead.

Now if we consider that we are surrounded by these energies at all times and imagine that we could see them we would see a dense web of energy forces radiating around us, influencing us.

This web carries forces that can impact many of us, and remedies made from imponderables add effective options for your homeopath.

For example, I have used the remedy So I made from the sun's rays to treat sunburn on many occasions with excellent results.

78. How are the remedies administered?

Usually the remedies are administered as pillules with instructions on how and when to take them.

71

They must be placed in a clean mouth under the tongue and allowed to dissolve over a few minutes. The remedies should not be touched by hand and nothing should be eaten or drunk for fifteen minutes before or fifteen minutes after taking the remedy.

79. What do I need to avoid while taking the remedy?

Coffee and mint should be avoided while taking the remedy.

80. Can I eat and drink with the remedy?

You will need to wait for fifteen minutes before and fifteen minutes after taking the remedy to eat or drink.

81. What if I can't take pills, is there another way?

Yes, the remedies can be made up in a liquid form as drops or in a powdered form to be poured onto the tongue.

82. Is there alcohol in the remedies?

There is a minute amount of alcohol in the remedies. The medicating bottle which is used to medicate the pills you will get is usually ninety percent alcohol. However, when a few drops are added to a bottle of hundreds of pillules, there is almost a negligible amount of alcohol in the remedy you receive as most of the alcohol evaporates instantly.

83. I can't take alcohol, can I still have a remedy?

It depends on your reason for not being able to have alcohol. Some people feel the effects of even the most tiny amount of alcohol and others may know that alcohol aggravates their symptoms. Recovering alcoholics do not want contact with alcohol at all as it may trigger cravings again and there are others who have severe chemical sensitivities and worry about coming into contact with alcohol.

Generally, when the medicating potency is added to pills, the alcohol evaporates in a few moments. However, there are methods that your homeopath can adopt to help you get the remedy without alcohol if necessary.

84. Is there sugar in the remedies?

Homeopaths use a variety of pillules and tablets. The tablets are a mix of lactose and sucrose. The pillules and granules are made from sucrose. Soft tablets made from lactose only are used when needed to dissolve very quickly.

85. I can't have sugar, can I still have a remedy?

Yes, as it can be made from lactose only tablets or made up as a liquid remedy

86. Can I touch the pills?

I advise not to touch the pills as they are surface coated. Most drugs produced have the chemical inside with a capsule or coating around it. With homeopathic pills, the medicated potency is dropped onto the pills. I advise using a teaspoon or tipping the pill into the lid of the bottle and then straight into your mouth. You soon get the knack!

**Do I need to change my lifestyle for it to work?**

87. Do I need to make other life changes for homeopathy to work?

Today, I doubt you will find any homeopath who will refuse to treat you unless you adopt all kinds of lifestyle changes, but we all know prevention is better than cure and so these changes may happen as a result of your improvement. So many lifestyle changes are simple, practical and available. So why not start with these: walking, breathing fresh air, meditating, being out in nature or whatever makes your heart sing.

Try to make sure you get good restorative sleep on a regular basis.

88. What about nutrition?

*'A man will spend the first half of his life ruining his health, and the second half searching for a cure'.*

Leonardo da Vinci

This is so important. Our bodies need the correct fuel to function correctly and we should also enjoy our food.

We should remember to eat a wide variety of whole foods, eat the right quantities to be a healthy weight and avoid sugar and additives as well.

We need to check that we are getting all the vitamins and minerals we need and if we drink alcohol, it should be to a sensible limit.

You may have heard about the microbiome recently, or about gut health in general. As the majority of hormones are produced in the gut as well as inflammation starting here, it is of vital importance that we look after our guts.

For more see:
http://pollytomlinson.co.uk/Gut%20Health.html

Personally, I believe keeping the body in an alkaline state helps to keep us well so if that can be achieved then that's great too. And remember to drink lots of water to keep our body's cells cleansed and hydrated.

89. What about movement and exercise?

*'Man sacrifices his health in order to make money. Then sacrifices money to recuperate his health'.*

Dalai Lama

The human body is designed to move and if it doesn't then things start to go wrong. Not many of us have jobs that involve exercise nowadays and so it is even more important to build some exercise and movement into our lifestyles. It is fairly easy to change habits to incorporate more walking, take the stairs not the lift for example.

We all need to exercise in some way which can include walking, for at least thirty minutes or more a day. This will improve your health significantly as your breathing and posture will improve, as will your cardiovascular health, your muscles and your skeletal system.

Aim to sweat through exercise at least twice a week.

90. What about my mindset?

This is such an important part of health and it will be addressed by your homeopath during the consultation. You may wish to discuss your feelings including anger, worry, stress, fear or you might be craving some quiet time away from the hustle and bustle of life. You may need to strengthen your deeply held beliefs or let go of those that no longer serve you.

91. What about my relationships?

Healthy relationships are so important to us humans. You may want to ask yourself if you have a strong network of friends, do you attend social gatherings with others, do you have at least one close friend to talk to, do you receive or give affection regularly and do you have any relatives that live close by? These are all things we should consider for ourselves especially as loneliness is so prevalent.

**Evidence and Research About Homeopathy**

92. Which epidemics have successfully been treated in the world using homeopathy?

Let me give you a few examples from the many over the last 200 years here:

In 1854 the London Homeopathic Hospital was turned over to cholera victims due to the epidemic. In this epidemic 54,000 people died. Under allopathic methods the death rate was 59.2% and under homeopathic treatment was just 16.4%.

In 1918 there was a Spanish Flu epidemic in America. Dr. T A McCann, from Dayton, Ohio reported that 24,000 cases of flu treated allopathically had a mortality rate of 28.2% while 26,000 cases of flu treated homoeopathically had a mortality rate of 1.05%.

This last figure was echoed and endorsed by Dr Dean W.A. Pearson of Philadelphia (Hahnemann

College) who recorded 26,795 cases of flu treated with homeopathy with the above result.

In 1975, Lathyrus was given to 30,000 – 40,000 [the number varies depending on the researcher reporting] individuals during a Buenos Aires polio epidemic, and not one of these patients reported contracting polio.

93. How many people use homeopathy in the world?

Over 500 million people use homeopathy worldwide.

94. How many people rely on homeopathy as their sole form of medicine?

Over 100 million people worldwide rely on homeopathy as their sole form of medicine.

95. Do the British Royal family use homeopathy?

Yes, they do, certainly Queen Elizabeth II and Prince Charles, *'... it is rooted in ancient traditions that intuitively understood the need to maintain balance and harmony with our minds, bodies, and the natural world'.*

The Queen Mother took homeopathy and maybe this contributed to her living for over 101 years.

In 1980, Ainsworths Homeopathic Pharmacy in London was honoured with Royal Warrants of Appointment to HM The Queen, HM The Queen Mother and HRH The Prince of Wales as suppliers of homeopathic remedies and have since earned a worldwide reputation as a centre of excellence.

96. Who else will I know who uses homeopathy?

Many celebrities use homeopathy and advocate its uses including Sir Paul McCartney, *'I can't manage without homeopathy. I never go anywhere without homeopathic remedies. I use them often'.*

Usain Bolt, *'I've been coming here since I was 16. It's been a long relationship. Every time I have a problem, he always gives me good advice and treatments'.*

Cher, *'I don't think I'd still be around today if it weren't for homeopathic medicine. I was sick with an Epstein-Barr virus which led to chronic fatigue and I couldn't work effectively for two years. I turned to a Sikh homeopathic doctor, almost in desperation. He started doing homeopathic stuff with herbs and vitamin therapy. Many doctors didn't believe in all that back then. Within four months, he'd got me up and back on the road again'.*

Kim Cattrall, *'Arnica! I love it! I use it all the time because I bruise easily'.*

Cindy Crawford, *'I am the doctor of our family and I'm a big fan of homeopathy. I always make sure I have it on me or in the medical kit. It works'.*

Others include Axl Rose, Moby, George Harrison, Pete Townsend, Victoria Beckham, Jennifer Aniston, Hillary and Bill Clinton, David Beckham and Tina Turner.

97. Why is homeopathy so controversial?

Homeopathic medicine is made from extremely small quantities of nanoparticles of substances extracted from plants, animals or minerals. The remedies are so diluted that, based on chemistry, it is difficult to find any molecules of the original substance in the remedy. This has led skeptics to speculate that there is nothing in a homeopathic remedy except water, implying that homeopathy cannot work.

98. Why is homeopathy negatively portrayed in the media?

It would appear that the skeptics have missed the point on how homeopathy works and as such feel the need to maintain their case against the efficacy of homeopathy.

However, this does not affect the great work that homeopaths do and will continue to do as science continues to discover the secrets of this science.

Nobel Prize-winning scientist, emeritus professor of Cambridge University Dr Brian Josephson said:

*'Simple-minded analysis may suggest that water, being a fluid, cannot have a structure of the kind that such a picture would demand. But cases such as that of liquid crystals, which while flowing like an ordinary fluid can maintain an ordered structure over macroscopic distances, show the limitations of such ways of thinking. There have not, to the best of my knowledge, been any refutations of homeopathy that remain valid after this particular point is taken into account'.*

99. What is the evidence that homeopathy works?

In 1991, three professors from the Netherlands who were not homeopaths, carried out a meta- analysis of 25 years of clinical studies using homeopathic medicines. They published the results in the British Medical Journal stating that of the 105 trials with results they could use, 81 indicated positive results. They found that 13 of 19 trials showed successful treatment of respiratory infections, 6 of 7 trials showed positive results in treating other infections, 5 of 7 trials showed improvement in diseases of the digestive system, 5 of 5 showed successful treatment of hay fever, 5 of 7 showed faster recovery after abdominal surgery, 4 of 6 promoted healing in treating rheumatological disease, 18 of 20 showed benefit in addressing pain or trauma, 8 of 10 showed positive results in relieving mental or psychological problems, and 13 of 15 showed benefit from miscellaneous diagnoses.

A body of clinical research in homeopathy that has been consistently recognised as some of the highest quality scientific research has been conducted by a group of researchers at the University of Glasgow and Glasgow Homeopathic Hospital. They conducted four studies on people suffering from various respiratory allergies (hay fever, asthma, and perennial allergic rhinitis). In total, they treated 253 patients and found a 28% improvement in visual analogue scores in those given a homeopathic medicine, as compared with a 3% improvement in patients given a placebo.

Three separate studies of children with diarrhoea were also conducted and published in scientific journals. A meta-analysis of the 242 children who were involved in these three studies showed that the children who were prescribed a homeopathic medicine experienced a highly significant reduction in the duration of diarrhoea, as compared with the children who were given a placebo.

One other study was on 53 patients with fibromyalgia. The participants were given individually chosen homeopathic treatment and showed significantly greater improvements in tender point count and tender point pain, quality of life, global health and a trend toward less depression compared with those on placebo.

What was also very interesting about this last trial was that the individuals receiving homeopathic treatment also experienced changes in their EEG readings. So, not only did the health of these people improve, but there were observable changes in brain activity.

This is very strong evidence that homeopathy can have observable effects.

100.Why do people believe it works if there is no scientific proof?

Medicines are usually tested using random controlled trials or RCTs. However, it is difficult to scientifically prove homeopathy using this method for a few reasons.

First, as we know now, the homeopathic remedy selected is chosen for the individual. RCTs are based on giving the same treatment to a large number of people and looking at the results compared to a control group who will have been given a placebo. As you have now learned, giving a large number of people the same remedy as they have the same general illness e.g. asthma, will not be appropriate in homeopathic terms as they would need their homeopath to select their correct individual remedy and their correct potency as no two people have the exact same symptoms.

This makes it very difficult to reflect whether a particular remedy is effective.

The second problem is that in an RCT, neither the patient nor the practitioner is supposed to know who is getting the placebo and who is getting the active treatment. In homeopathic treatment the homeopath needs to observe the individual's reaction to the first remedy to enable them to decide how to proceed. If there has been no reaction, the homeopath would know that the wrong remedy or potency had been given but only if they knew a remedy had been given in the first place.

Again, this makes it very difficult to reflect on whether the particular remedy has been effective.

101. Who are the scientists working towards further proof of homeopath's efficacy?

Dr Luc Montagnier is a Nobel Prize-winning virologist who supports homeopathy.

He has been researching how the electromagnetic signals of an original medicine remain in water after a sequence of dilution and vigorous shaking in between each dilution has taken place. Dr Montagnier's research shows that the water undergoes biological effects.

*'I can't say that homeopathy is right in everything. What I can say now is that the high dilutions (used in homeopathy) are right. High dilutions of something are not nothing. They are water structures which mimic the original molecules'.*

Nobel Prize-winning scientist, emeritus professor of Cambridge University Dr Brian Josephson wrote this in response to an article about Homeopathy in New Scientist:

*'Regarding your comments on claims made for homeopathy: criticisms centred around the vanishingly small number of solute molecules present in a solution after it has been repeatedly diluted are beside the point, since advocates of homeopathic remedies attribute their effects not to molecules present in the water, but to modifications of the water's structure'.*

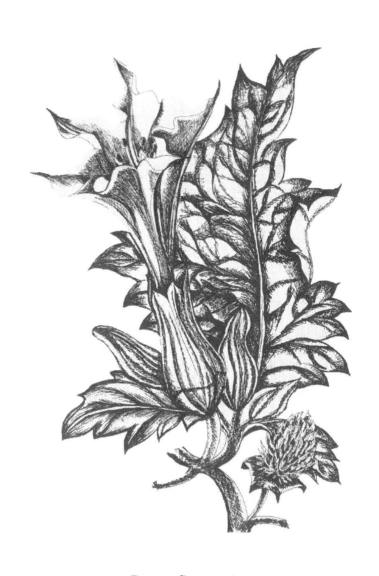

*Datura Stramonium*

## Chapter *4*

# So, What Have You Learned from This Book?

From reading this book, so far you may have been introduced to a new way of thinking about health and dis-ease in the body. You have been introduced to a way of understanding how your body may behave when it is out of balance. You have been introduced to a complimentary medicine which yields results and has good quality studies to prove its effectiveness. You have been introduced to the idea that using less drug therapy will improve your immune system and not only reduce your chances of becoming ill in the future but also help you to get better right now.

As human beings, we should all have the right to choose how we look after ourselves and if we choose to do this using natural means then this should be available to us. The use of complimentary medicine in my view is a way of keeping ourselves and those of our loved ones in the best health we can whilst also standing up for our freedom of choice. We should be able to stand up and shout for the type of health care we want generally.

My intention for writing this book was to raise awareness of homeopathy as although it is used by millions of people worldwide, this still only accounts for approximately 10% of the UK population. I am very happy that the use of homeopathy is on the increase once again. It is a positive sign that people such as yourself are ready to look for healthy alternatives once again in light of their awareness being raised to side effects and the failure of drugs to actually work for them.

It is my firm belief that more complimentary and alternative medicines will become available to all in the future as the public awareness grows. You will already be aware of many of the problems associated with the conventional medicine approach to health and there is now far more support for natural alternative choices from the public, therapists and medics alike. It seems to me that the time is now to embrace a holistic approach to health, where all aspects of your life are taken into consideration and not just the part that is deemed to need fixing. We must develop bespoke treatment for each individual and find ways to live healthier, wholehearted lives.

I also believe that we should all work on ourselves. If we each approach our own health as individuals and look for the natural ways to improve our health and lifestyles, then the overall impact could be extremely powerful. Homeopathy is one of the deepest and effective ways of healing that I have experienced and its energy is very potent. It opens the door to a journey into health that is complete and permanent and this is very exciting.

On a practical level, the use of homeopathy as a whole will reduce the number of drugs prescribed and therefore make the use of some drugs more effective should the time arise when they are truly needed. Natural remedies do not create resistant strains and there are so many reasons to learn about alternatives to drugs.

Benjamin Franklin said, 'An ounce of prevention is worth a pound of cure'.

I hope that through reading this book, you can appreciate both the need for safer alternatives as well as the passion I have for homeopathy to become more and more available to you. I have told you how homeopathy can treat simple infections such as coughs, bronchitis, throat and ear infections amongst numerous other chronic and auto immune diseases.

All that is needed from you is an open mind to treating illness.

You have been introduced to something here that may challenge your beliefs. I would ask you to look at the data available if you're interested, and consider homeopathy as another viable means of treating illnesses rather than with drugs. Think of the effects we could have on the health of everyone globally if we all took less antibiotics for example and used homeopathy.

You now know that people who use homeopathy alongside conventional medicine have much better outcomes, using less drugs, costing less and with fewer side effects. The effect of us all using just one less drug would be enormous.

These remedies still work, there are so many non-drug solutions to infections and illnesses. I hope that now you are ready to learn what your alternatives are and how to take action.

You have learned about homeopathy, how it works and how safe it is. I have introduced you to the philosophy and history of homeopathy. Hopefully I have answered your questions about whether homeopathy is for you and what to expect from it. And you have been told about lifestyle changes that you may need to implement to achieve optimum health. You have also been told about the ongoing research and evidence to support homeopathy, this is an exciting area of research.

Perhaps you are a parent and you would like to see your child grow with a strong and healthy immune system. To not have your little one's body subjected to the onslaught of drugs from almost the second they are born. Perhaps you would like them to stay as pure and strong as possible and to have far less illness growing up as a result of an amazingly strong and robust body and non-compromised immune system.

Or perhaps you have an illness yourself and you are fed up with the drug regime and the side effects. Maybe you're not feeling any better and your physician has no positive news for you. Let me ask you, what have you got to lose? If you are ready to consider an alternative or ready to try homeopathy alongside your conventional medicine to begin with then go for it!

Would you like to feel happy, amazing, vibrant, full of energy and symptom-free without side effects?

I know most people would. Then it's time for you to take action and contact me for advice. Having all this knowledge is great but you need to take action today rather than procrastinating any longer. Make today your Day 1 rather than saying 1 Day!

*'Homeopathy cures a larger percentage of cases than any other method of treatment and is beyond doubt safer and more economical and the complete medical science'.*

Mahatma Gandhi

Why don't you begin by considering the toxicity in your life and begin by reducing this as best you can? Start today with the chemical toxins that are around you, this is a good place to begin. Then let me help you with the internal, emotional and bacterial, viruses and fungi that need to be eliminated.

Toxins are varied and many. A broad category of toxins includes:

Chemical: External, e.g. Insecticides, household cleaners, cosmetics, soap, toothpaste, additives, drugs, vaccines, chemicals in water, air pollutants etc.

Internal: i.e. made in the body, e.g. increased adrenalin, hormones, dead cells etc.

Hereditary/Genetic

Emotional: stress, worry, anxiety, anger, insult etc.

Perverse Energy: electromagnetic, electricity, geopathic radiation (from computers, mobile phones, TV's, X-rays, aeroplanes, power lines etc.)

Bacteria/Viruses/Parasites/Fungi

The other thing you could consider right now is any deficiencies. Ask yourself about your nutrition, exercise, sunlight, water, rest and love. Are there any small changes you could begin with here? I can assist with your nutrition and encourage you with your new regimes.

Think about adequate water intake, adequate exercise, meditation, looking at relationships, working hours and possibly your living environment.

When I work with you, we will look at these matters with a view to finding a life balance.

Contact me through my website www.pollytomlinson.co.uk or through Facebook Messenger.

Here is the link to my Facebook page: https://www.facebook.com/pollysremedies/ and you can also follow me on Instagram here: https://www.instagram.com/pollytomlinson/?hl=en

Please remember the journey to good health is a process. Getting well is not about taking or doing ONE thing. It involves a certain amount of commitment on your part.

**IT IS NOT ALWAYS EASY, BUT IT IS ALWAYS WORTH IT!!**

# *Chapter* **5**

## It's Time to Take Action

So now you know that there is a safe, effective alternative to that which you already know. An alternative that has no side effects and is proven to work, what do you do now?

Knowledge is amazing, but without applying the knowledge it becomes worthless.

*'Each time a (person) stands up for an ideal, or acts to improve the lot of others...he sends forth a tiny ripple of hope, and crossing each other from a million different centres of energy and daring those ripples build a current that can sweep down the mightiest walls of oppression and resistance...'.*

Robert F Kennedy

If anything you have read has moved you or touched you in any way then I would urge you to get in touch with myself, a fully qualified and registered homeopath to help you and your loved ones with the ailments you have now.

Here's what I'm going to offer you in return for the time you have invested in reading this book: I'm offering you a 15-minute call to find out if homeopathy can help you. I am aware that some people resist contacting a homeopath as there is a cost involved immediately and I would like to remove this obstacle to even finding out if Homeopathy could help you. Other homeopaths charge for this but I would like to waive this initial charge as you have invested time in this book.

So, if you would like to receive this free 15-minute call then please email me at polly@homeopathy101.co.uk with the subject heading FREE PRELIMINARY CONSULTATION and I will send you a link to book in. It's that easy.

Please also connect with me for more information via my website www.pollytomlinson.co.uk

I would invite you to connect/follow me on social media

https://www.facebook.com/pollysremedies/

https://www.instagram.com/pollytomlinson/?hl=en

And take positive steps today towards a brighter future for yourself, your family and friends and globally.

It would also be fantastic if those of you who have read the book leave a review, or buy a copy of the book for a friend or family member or recommend it to those who may need it today.

# Links and References

Ainsworths Pharmacy: https://www.ainsworths.com

Helios Pharmacy: https://www.helios.co.uk

The Homeopathic Supply Company:
http://www.hsconline.co.uk/home

The Alliance of Registered Homeopaths: www.a-r-h.org

Crockett, P. (1995) The Unfolded Organon, A Precis of Hahnemann's Sixth Edition

Professor Jacques Benveniste, (1988) Nature. (Nature 1988;333: 816-8 [PubMed])

Johnson, C.M. (2012) Good Medicine: Homeopathy. Available at https://www.bmj.com/content/345/bmj.e6184/rr/616928

Extraordinary Medicine (2017) Homeopathy: A History of Opposition. Available at http://extraordinarymedicine.org

Integrated Medicine Institute (2017) What's in the Little White Balls? Homeopathy Explained.

Available at https://www.imi.com.hk/what-s-in-the-little-white-balls.html

The Hahnemann College of Homeopathy:
http://www.hchuk.com

The School of Shamanic Homeopathy:
http://www.shamanic-homoeopathy.com

Your Health, Your Choice (2017) Why a Nobel Prize winning doctor supports homeopathy. Available at:
https://www.yourhealthyourchoice.com.au/news-features/why-nobel-prize-winning-doctor-supports-homeopathy/

16167299R00057

Printed in Great Britain
by Amazon